WHOLEY COW

A SIMPLE GUIDE TO EATING AND LIVING

BARBARA RODGERS

TABLE OF CONTENTS

ACKNOWLEDGMENTS

First of all I would like to thank God for giving me the divine inspiration and guidance to write this book and for His ever present love.

I would like to thank my family for your love and support. You all mean the world to me and am so grateful to have you in my life.

- To husband, Chris, you are the love of my life and a wonderful father to our children and amazing person. Thank you for your friendship, caring and being my soul-mate.
- To my daughter, Angela, thank you for giving me useful tips and inspiring suggestions for the book. You are creative and smart, and I appreciate your knowledge.
- To my daughter, Sara, thank you for doing the cover design for the book and giving your time and energy into developing sketches. You are creative and talented, and I appreciate your help in making this idea and project become a reality.

I would like to extend a special thank you to Maria Rafdal, L.Ac.
http://rafdalacu.com/

Maria is a licensed acupuncturist with a master's degree in Oriental Medicine (MSOM) from Southwest Acupuncture College in Boulder, CO and has focused training in women's health.

Thank you, Maria, for confirming women have alternative choices when it comes to their health.

Thank you for your knowledge, caring, compassion and support. I am forever grateful you confirmed what my intuition told me.

Thanks also goes out to Jake Sweete, LAc., MSAc., LMT.
https://cloudmountainanalects.com/

Jake is a licensed acupuncturist and trained with some of the most well-respected Chinese Medicine practitioners and scholars in the United States.

Thank you, Jake, for your wisdom, caring, compassion, inspiration and sweet personality. Your help is greatly appreciated.

INTRODUCTION

INTRODUCTION

If you've picked up this book, you probably know there is an obesity epidemic in this country and countless people who have health issues related to their diets, but...

Wholey Cow!

How did we get here and, more importantly, what can you do about it?

That is a question many people are asking. While there are hundreds of different diets out there to try, it is no longer a question of which one will work or which exercise program to follow. We need to look at what we are eating and calling food and the whole food supply system. If you look back in time, it is easy to see how food has changed, especially over the last 50 years. It is amazing how food has grown and evolved. Even in my own experience, I can see how food has changed and evolved, and I am sure if you think about, you can too.

My Story

I was raised in a family with six kids, where meals were an integral part of our family life. From early on, we were all expected to help out around the house with meal preparation, setting the table, cleaning up and other family chores. Looking back, our meals seemed pretty basic to me and seemed to consist of the same old things: cereal, pop tarts or eggs for breakfast; a sandwich, soup or macaroni and cheese for lunch; and supper, as we called it, always included some sort of meat, potatoes and a vegetable.

Sometimes we would have fruit or another sweet treat for dessert. We played outside when not in school and drank water from our garden hose when thirsty. Like other kids in the neighborhood, we drank Kool Aid, but didn't have it every day. Soda pop was considered a treat and something we had only on special occasions.

By the time I reached junior high, I remember a shift in our eating pattern. My older brothers had jobs or were in sports and weren't around for supper as much. It seemed like we started to eat more varieties of food, as more processed food started appearing at the grocery store. It didn't take long to talk our mom into buying frozen pizzas and other processed foods, as they were convenient, easy to make and cheap to buy. By the time I reached high school, diet soda pop had become all the rage. I am not sure how I did it, but somehow I talked my mom into buying diet soda pop on a consistent basis. It was sugar-free and all of my friends were drinking it. We drank Tab, Diet Pepsi, and Diet Coke. We couldn't seem to get enough and often downed it with a bag of red licorice. Yikes! This was the start of a thirty-some year addiction to diet soda pop for me. It wasn't until around my 50th birthday that I decided to give up my morning Diet Coke. It was time to take a hard look at my diet. I personally never had issues with weight, but was starting to have some health concerns. It was then I realized food is something more than what you put in your mouth that tastes good. It is an energy source for your body, containing specific nutrients and information vital for maintaining health.

It was December 2013, less than a month until my 50th birthday, and I never remembered feeling so down. I wasn't sure what happened and why I was feeling so unhappy.

The holidays were just around the corner and I typically loved the joyous Christmas season. This year was different. My family was planning a party for my upcoming birthday and although I should have been excited, I felt nothing except dread. It wasn't the fact I was turning 50. I knew 50 was just a number and you are as young as you feel, but I was feeling old. I was run-down, had no energy, and couldn't concentrate.

I lost my wedding ring the month before and was unhappy about it, but there was more to it. I wasn't myself and hadn't been for a while. I remember going to work and just staring at my computer. I have always been a high-energy person and go-getter, so this was strange. On top of everything, I noticed my hair had been falling out over the last year, and it was more than a couple strands in the shower. Thankfully, God blessed me with thick hair so no one noticed except me. At first, I thought the hair loss was hormonal and possibly related to perimenopause. As my hair got thinner, though, I was determined to figure out why.

What is perimenopause?

Perimenopause:
The time leading up to menopause (can be 10-15 years prior) when estrogen and other hormone levels in a woman's body start to fluctuate and decline. Various symptoms can occur, including irregular and heavy bleeding, hot flashes, night sweats, anxiety, sleep problems, mood swings, irritability, weight gain and more. Symptoms can vary among women and are very individual, so there is often confusion and angst at this time. While many women are symptomatic, not all women are affected by perimenopause.[1]

In January 2014, my energy level hit an all-time low and all I wanted to do was sleep. I knew something wasn't right. Then it dawned on me—maybe the hair loss and low-energy had something to do with the iron level in my body. I decided to do a Google search and up came multiple articles on iron deficiency anemia.

DID YOU KNOW?
Iron deficiency anemia affects more people than any other condition.[2]

> **What is iron deficiency anemia?**
>
> *Iron deficiency anemia:*
> A condition where your blood lacks adequate healthy red blood cells. It typically is caused by an insufficient amount of iron in the body and can result from numerous different causes, including lack of iron in your diet, iron absorption issues, or blood loss in the body from an ulcer, polyp, cancer or some other illness. It can also be caused by heavy periods in women, especially during perimenopause. Without enough iron, the body can't produce hemoglobin, which helps carry oxygen throughout the body and a multitude of symptoms can occur including fatigue, disorientation, memory issues, moodiness, irritability, depression, hair loss, anxiety and sleepiness.[3]

As I read through the articles, I was convinced this was causing my symptoms, so I made a doctor's appointment to find out for sure. After my visit and a number of blood tests, my suspicions were confirmed. My iron stores were practically depleted. My ferritin test was super low (2.5 to be exact).

> **What is ferritin?**
>
> *Ferritin:*
> "A blood cell protein.
>
> *Ferritin Test:*
> A ferritin test measures the amount of iron your body is storing. If your ferritin level is low, your iron stores are low, indicating you have iron deficiency .
>
> *Normal ferritin range for men:*
> 20 to 500 nanograms per milliliter (standard units).
>
> *Normal ferritin range for women:*
> 20 to 200 nanograms per milliliter (standard units)."[4]

That explains why I wasn't feeling like myself. Needless to say, my body needed time to recuperate. My doctor prescribed iron supplements and suggested I eat an iron-rich diet. I followed the recommendations, yet

was curious why I developed an iron deficiency in the first place.
I felt compelled to learn more about nutrition, and after doing a little online research, I stumbled upon the Institute for Integrative Nutrition®, a well-known nutrition school, and decided to enroll.

In the program I learned over 100 different dietary theories, as well as a variety of coaching techniques. Additionally, I discovered the importance of self-care and how eating better can help eliminate many ailments. Along the way, I discovered some commonalities found in many diets.

This book is about what I learned on my journey back to health. It includes 7 guiding principles anyone can use to help restore health, well-being and wholeness to life.

If you are wondering about the title of the book, I decided to call it *Wholey Cow* because whole foods became important to me on my journey and beef is a good source for iron (especially if you are battling iron deficiency or iron deficiency anemia).

WHOLE FOOD

In The Beginning

In The Beginning

"Then God said, 'Behold, I have given you every plant yielding seed that is on the surface of all the earth and every tree which has fruit yielding seed; it shall be food for you; and to every beast of the earth and to every bird of the sky and to everything that moves on the earth which has life, I have given every green plant for food and it was so.'"
—Genesis 1:29-30

From the beginning of time, God provided everything we need to eat and live. From the Old Testament to the New Testament, there are countless passages in the bible referring to food and well-being. Fruits, vegetables, grains and spices are some foods referenced. Meat is also mentioned including fish, fowl and the cow, which was considered sacred. Calves were often used as sacrificial offerings and served only at special feasts. These foods provided sustenance and life energy. But why do we eat so differently today?

That answer is complicated and involves problems created on many levels from industrialization, factory farming and big business. Lobbyists for drug companies and farmers press the government to make decisions affecting our well-being and the food supply. People living in biblical times worked and ate from the land and sea. Many people today eat from a box, a bag or drive-thru, and some are still asking, "Where's the beef?"

One thing is clear—our food system needs reform. Society today con-sumes more processed food containing artificial preservatives and ingredients than real, wholesome foods. It's bizarre. Many people don't know the difference and think "food is just food" and therein lies part of the problem. Many of us are eating the wrong foods. Eating too much processed food and the wrong kinds of food can cause weight gain and illness.

DID YOU KNOW?

*Over 65% of Americans are overweight and
almost half the population has a chronic disease.[5]*

Many people turn to fad-diets to lose weight. What most people really need is a diet over-haul! People often look for a quick-fix for a growing waistline or a medical problem. Fad diets, although popular, often only offer a temporary solution. A life-style change that improves eating habits is a better solution.

Someone mentioned to me once they wanted to try the cabbage soup diet to lose a few pounds. I thought to myself, "the cabbage soup diet, are you serious?" If I had to follow this diet, I'd probably go a little crazy, even if it was only for a few weeks or few days. It is easy to see how people gain weight back. I'm sure you've heard of the "yo-yo" diet affect. It is not hard to figure out where the term came from. After doing a deprivation diet, your taste buds naturally scream for variety. In addition, your body is practically starving for nutrients. Eating whole foods is the best way to supply nutrients for bodily functions. Most processed foods, on the other hand, contain merely a few vitamins and minerals, and many are loaded with chemicals and preservatives.

In Loma Linda, California, there's a Blue Zone area where people live longer, healthier lives than most others around the world. It is ironic, but people in this area follow a diet reflecting what God intended for us all in the story of the Garden of Eden. In fact, there's a large American epidemiology study done that shows this type of diet to be one of the healthiest available to human-kind today. This Blue Zone diet consists largely of beans and raw vegetables. Cooked vegetables are part of this diet too, including asparagus, broccoli and cabbage. People in this Blue Zone also enjoy nuts and dates for a simple dessert.[6]

> **What is a Blue Zone?**
>
> **Blue Zone:**
> Regions found in different parts of the world with the longest living cultures and the most living Centarians (people over 100 years in age). People living in Blue Zones live long, healthy lives by combining a healthy diet of whole foods with a healthy life style. People in Blue Zones tend to have low stress, strong connected communities and healthy, loving relationships with family and friends. Moderate exercise is part of their daily lives.[7]

This way of eating sounds a lot healthier than the way many of us eat today. Did you notice no processed foods were mentioned in the diet? It is easy to see why people in this Blue Zone are among the healthiest in the world. Whole foods and whole living—this sounds like a good plan for us all. Following are seven principles to eat well and live well.

PRINCIPLE #1

FOOD IS FUEL

Food Is Fuel

"Let food be thy medicine and medicine be thy food."
—Hippocrates

You may have heard the saying, "Food is Fuel," but how many people really take it to heart and feed their body the information and nutrients it needs? Sadly, not many of us do. That's not surprising, as people today no longer pay much attention to eating for sustenance. Instead, many of us look for good tasting, easy to prepare food. Most processed foods, nonetheless, are loaded with preservatives to give them a long shelf-life. Who knows what effect these additives really have on your body? We have become lab rats for food companies and no one knows the exact outcome.

Your body needs a variety of nutrients to produce skin, muscle, hair, finger nails, bone and more. Moreover, it needs nutrients for your blood to carry oxygen to all parts of the body and to carry out hosts of other bodily functions. Most nutrients you need come from fruits, vegetables, whole grains, nuts, seeds and meat. Our society over the years has turned away from a lot of these foods and that is a problem. Whole foods tend to be more expensive and aren't as convenient as many processed food items. Many consumers look for food products that cost less and take minimal work to prepare. Years ago, children were taught at an early age how to cook and were involved in the process. This doesn't happen as much today. Many of us are busy running from work to a child's sporting event or this meeting or that meeting and don't have the time or energy to prepare a home-cooked meal. Many people find it easier to opt for a frozen pizza, go out to eat or prepare some other packaged food item.

Processed foods may contain some nutrients your body needs, but definitely not the same amount or the quality you get when you eat whole foods. For example, let's take a look at the apple. The apple is considered to be one of the healthier foods available. Apples are rich in vitamin C and contain a fair amount of fiber. They have other healthful benefits and nutrients, like magnesium, vitamin B-6, iron, vitamin A and calcium. When you compare this to apple sauce, a processed version of an apple, you might find the content of vitamin C to be about the same or maybe higher, but the fiber content is lower. Other nutrients originally present in the apple might be missing. The apple sauce might contain added ingredients, such as high fructose corn syrup or another sweetener. This depends on the brand you are looking at, but have you ever wondered why the processed version has more ingredients? Obviously, a certain amount of ingredients are added to obtain a longer shelf life. Others may be added to make the product look a certain way. The bottom line is you should examine what you eat. The next time you are out grocery shopping, take a hard look at the food you are selecting. Perhaps you will make better choices if you open your eyes wider?

Fortified Foods

There are a number of reasons processed foods contain different ingredients than whole foods. Packaged foods may contain a number of whole food ingredients, yet the original nutrients and vitamins are often stripped out during processing. To make up for this, foods are frequently fortified.

What is fortification?

Fortification:
A process where nutrients are added to a food product where it did not naturally occur.[8]

A few examples of fortification include adding vitamin D to milk, calcium to orange juice or adding omega-3 fatty acids to eggs. Fortification is a common practice and is supported by both the World Health Organization (WHO) and the Food and Agricultural Organization of the United Nations. It is used to intentionally increase the essential micronutrients in foods whether they were originally there before processing or not. Fortification is used to improve the nutrient quality of foods with minimal public risk to health.[9] In fact, according to Project Healthy Children (PHC), "Fortification is a safe, effective way to improve public health and has been used throughout the world since the 1920s. Some common fortified foods include staples such as salt, maize flour, wheat flour, sugar, vegetable oil and rice."[10] Other common fortified foods include cereals, milk, breads and eggs, as well as a host of other packaged foods.

When out grocery shopping, you might notice foods fortified with the mineral iron. These products are important for individuals with low-iron and iron deficiency anemia, or those who want to maintain a certain iron level in their body. A few examples of foods fortified with iron are Raisin Bran and other cereals, as well as most bread products. Additionally, people looking to increase their calcium intake to perhaps build or maintain strong, healthy bones, may be drawn to products fortified with calcium.

Enriched Foods

In addition to fortification, a variety of food products are enriched with nutrients. Sometimes when a food is processed, some vitamins and minerals are lost and then added back. Some examples of enriched foods are flour, bread and pasta noodles.

What are enriched foods?

Enriched Foods:
Enriched food products have nutrients added back in that were removed or lost during processing.[11]

DID YOU KNOW?

Approximately 12% of non-Hispanic white women, 50% of pregnant women and 2% of men are iron deficient.[12]

What Are We Really Eating?

Fortifying and enriching foods is not a bad thing and was developed to prevent malnutrition. The problem is our society consumes way too many processed foods today, whether they are fortified and enriched or not. Many of these processed foods contain chemicals and preservatives, along with added sugars, artificial sweeteners, processed fats, high fructose corn syrup and more. These additives and preservatives can wreak havoc on your body. If you purchase an item to get more iron or calcium in your diet, you need to take a hard look at what else is in the product. Manufacturers often use gimmicks to get you to buy a product and may draw your attention to 1 or 2 nutrients in the product. Consumers are often swayed into buying these products because of the packaging claims. The end result is you might be buying unhealthy products, even though they have added nutrients.

Read Those Labels

One way to help prevent this is to read food labels. Most consumers, including myself, don't make a habit of reading food labels. When I needed to add more iron into my diet, however, reading packaging labels became very important. Overall, I ate pretty well, yet frequently over-looked the long list of ingredients on packaged foods. When is the last time you took a hard look at a food label? Did you notice the number of ingredients? How many of the ingredients could you pronounce? Do you know what they are? It is a little scary when you think about it.

Fat and sugar repeatedly top the food additive list. It's amazing how many products contain them in one form or another. Although you can try and educate yourself on the many names for sugar, fat and hard-to-pronounce ingredients, it's better to avoid them when possible.

A diet rich in whole foods is the best source of nutrients for your body. Many of these options come without packaging labels, as they are provided by Mother Nature. Remember—the fewer ingredients the better when buying food products.

Wholey Cow Tips:

1. Choose fruits, vegetables, whole grains, nuts, seeds and meat to get the most nutrients for your body.
2. Avoid food products containing ingredients you aren't familiar with, especially if there are a lot of them.
3. Be cautious about buying a food product with a specific packaging claim, such as fortified with extra calcium. Make sure you take the time to read all the ingredients in the product.
4. Start noticing and reading packaging labels.
5. Try to purchase food in its most simple state.

PRINCIPLE #2

KNOW THYSELF

Know Thyself

"Know yourself to improve yourself."
—Auguste Comte

Individuality

There are literally hundreds of diets out there for you to try—from low-carb to high-carb, low-fat to high-protein, the Atkins Diet, the Mediterranean Diet and the list goes on. Isn't it funny how some people have luck with one diet and others may not? Restrictive diets may work for some people. For others, cravings may be hard to avoid. Feelings can change over time too. Perhaps you wanted to avoid a certain food and all of sudden you no longer want to pass it up? It is hard to predict what may happen when there are restrictions. Diets can be confusing. Have you ever tried a diet and had good results, only to stop losing weight suddenly after a period of time? This can be frustrating and stressful. It is easy to see why you might go back to unhealthy eating patterns. Diets can have varying results and are very individual. But why is that?

That's an interesting question many doctors, dietitians and nutritionists have pondered over the years. There is an interesting viewpoint on this topic, called *bio-individuality*. This theory incorporates the idea that there's no one right diet that works for everyone all of the time.[13] We are all unique individuals who come from various ethnic backgrounds and upbringings. The theory of bio-individuality takes into account your ancestry, your blood type and your metabolic rate. All of these factors can have an effect on how you react to food.

Looking back, I grew up eating more of an ancestral diet. My ancestors are from Germany, so my family enjoyed hearty meals with a lot of meat and potatoes. In fact, I remember eating so much beef growing up that as I got older, I didn't much care for it. There was a period of time when I rarely ate it at all. It just didn't taste good to me anymore. Over the years, I ate much more chicken than beef and more salads than potatoes. This could be one reason I developed an iron deficiency. I wasn't including enough iron-rich beef in my diet. My body was literally craving "the cow" I grew up on.

I'm not surprised, as meat contains heme iron, which is more easily absorbed by the body than non-heme iron.

What is heme iron?

Heme iron:
Heme iron is found in animals and typically attached to proteins, called heme proteins.

Heme iron is the best source of iron for people who are iron deficient.

What is non-heme iron?

Non-Heme Iron: Non-heme iron is found in vegetables, grains and some processed foods. You can also find it in nuts, vegetables, fruit and iron supplements.[15]

Good sources of heme iron:

- Beef
- Chicken
- Oysters
- Clams
- Turkey
- Ham
- Veal
- Tuna
- Liver
- Salmon
- Eggs
- Shrimp
- Chicken Liver
- Mussels
- Lamb
- Sardines
- Pork Loin
- Halibut

Good sources of non-heme iron:

- Cereal
- Beans
- Bread
- Potatoes
- Noodles
- Rice
- Apricots
- Raisins
- Strawberries
- Spinach
- Kale
- Broccoli
- Pasta
- Nuts (almonds, cashews, etc.)
- Peas
- Oatmeal
- Molasses
- Tofu[16]

I now eat beef several times a week. It helps keep my iron and energy up and I enjoy the taste again. I look for good-quality cuts of beef and frequently opt for grass-fed beef selections.

Carnivore Vs. Omnivore

Opinions vary when it comes to eating meat. Adding more meat to my diet was a good choice given my ancestral background and need for iron. I know this is not the case for everyone. Many people are strongly opposed to eating meat and follow a vegetarian or a vegan diet. Other people may eat meat on occasion and still others may merely eat certain varieties. Again, it is a personal choice and should be respected, as there are pros and cons to both. If you eat meat, it should be in moderation. Most nutritionists agree a serving of meat should be the size of your fist. Yes—fist! Many restaurants would have you believing otherwise and many times they serve portions twice the size they should be. In reality, given our ancestry, over the last several decades consumers have been eating more meat than the body is accustomed to eating.

Grains Galore/Grain Free

Whole grains have been a central part of the human diet since early civilization. That is typical, as they are prevalent in many areas of the world. Grains are an excellent source of nutrients and help provide sustained energy for the body. Many grains contain iron, fiber, vitamin E, vitamin B and variety of other essential enzymes.

Although grains provide beneficial nutrients for your body, there is some controversy surrounding them these days. Grains have been around for thousands of years, but today's grains are much different and bear little resemblance to the grains in our diet thousands of years ago.[17]

Many grains today are genetically modified and are treated with chemicals to help preserve them and give them a longer shelf live.

What are genetically modified organisms?

Genetically Modified Organisms (GMOs):
Foods produced from organisms that have altered DNA due to the process of genetic engineering, a process which alters traits. Some common crops that are genetically modified include: soybeans, corn, cotton and canola.[18]

It's a small wonder some people have developed allergies, food sensitivities and issues with gluten as a result.

DID YOU KNOW?

An elimination diet can help identify foods you may be allergic or sensitive to, such as grains.

If you enjoy grains, there is quite a variety to choose from. Some common grains include wheat, rice and oats. Other alternate grains available are quinoa, buckwheat, couscous, barley, amaranth, millet, spelt and kamut. Several grains have gained more popularity recently, yet date back to biblical times. Grains today are abundant in supply and are found in a large variety of processed foods.

Grains are a staple in the diet of many consumers. They are easy to make and can be prepared in a variety of ways. Grains have a distinct texture and mild flavor. To enhance the flavor, you can add herbs, spices and vegetables. Grains work well as a side dish for lunch or dinner. They also can make a healthy breakfast choice. Try adding fruit, nuts, seeds, greens or avocados to your morning rice or quinoa.

Feast on Fats

When it comes to adding fat to your diet, some people are apprehensive. That is understandable, since there is a great deal of conflicting information on fat these days. The low-fat craze of the 90s is still stuck in the minds of many, causing confusion and skepticism. Fat became a bad word and something to avoid. Many food manufacturers latched on to this notion and developed hundreds of low-fat food products.

Although low-fat foods are popular, they aren't all healthy. Fat plays a big part in how a food tastes. When the fat content of a food is reduced or eliminated, something has to take its place. Sugar and artificial sweeteners are frequently added to the product to make it taste better than or similar to the original version. Chemicals and preservatives are regularly added along with sweeteners. Another area of concern with a low-fat diet is the thinking that we all need to reduce our fat intake to avoid problems with heart disease and cholesterol. This claim was never proven and corresponds with the belief that fat in general is bad for you. The problem with this thinking is most low-fat diets focus on the total fat of food.

A lot of people focusing on the fat content of food repeatedly avoid it altogether. This can be hard on your body and detrimental to certain body functions. Your body needs fat to aid in movement and perform peak functions. The key to fat intake is definitely not deprivation. Instead of focusing on low-fat, no fat or total fat, you need to look at the type of fat you are eating. Fats can be divided into two categories—good fats and bad fats. Both good fats and bad fats affect your body differently.

There are a variety of fats found in foods including saturated fat, monounsaturated fat, polyunsaturated fat and trans-fats. Monounsaturated fats (MUFAS), are the good fats and help your body function optimally. MUFAS are plant-based and are found in an assortment of whole foods. You can find them in avocados, nuts, seeds, olives and dark chocolate. Other healthy fats can be found in coconut oil, olive oil, grape seed oil, and a variety of fish.

Trans-fats, on the other hand, are not so good and can be found in some animals and animal products, like milk. Other trans-fats are man-made and are created by an industrialization process where vegetable oil is turned into a solid form. This type of oil is called partially hydrogenated oil and is found in many processed foods (think corn chips, potato chips, crackers and other boxed and bagged food products). Try and eliminate this type of fat from your diet or use it sparingly. Eat healthier fats when possible. A handful of nuts are a better choice versus a handful of potato chips.

Keep a Food Journal

Most people can easily describe what they like and dislike regarding the taste and texture of food. Describing how a particular food makes you feel, however, can be a different story. We live in a fast-paced society where many people literally eat and run, so this can be challenging. If you are rushed or focused on getting back to work or your child's soccer game, you're probably not going to notice how a slice of pizza made you feel. The headache or bloated feeling you have later in the day, on the other hand, could be attributed to the pizza and soda pop you had for lunch.

When is the last time you truly noticed how you felt after eating something? For many of us, the answer is probably not too often and for others, maybe never—which is kind of sad. It can be difficult to know how a food makes you feel if you don't check in with yourself on a regular basis.

Writing down what you eat is a great way to get to know yourself. Keeping a food journal can help uncover specific food habits, patterns and emotional triggers. Additionally, recording what you eat and how you feel can help you make better food choices. Use the information you record as your guide.

As an example, let's assume you tend to crave something sweet in the afternoon. One day you might choose a cookie for your afternoon snack.

Another day you may choose an apple. Most likely you will feel a little different when you choose an apple over a cookie. Both items are sweet and may give you a quick burst of energy. The cookie, conversely, might leave you feeling "icky" or a little "blue" later on. Keeping a food journal can help you discover some important information about the foods you are eating and how they affect you.

What is a food journal?

Food Journal:
A way to record what you eat, how the food makes you feel, etc. Food journals can be used to discover food allergies, eating patterns, emotional food triggers and more. Using a food journal is a powerful way to change food eating habits.

Following is some information you can record in a food journal:

1. Date
2. Time
3. Food consumed
4. Meal/snack
5. Emotion felt before eating
6. How hungry you were
7. Portion size
8. Exercise done for the day

Food Journal Options

There are many options when it comes to food journals. You can easily find one by Googling "food journals," or find an app for your phone. You can also create your own food journal using a spreadsheet or table. Use a notebook if you prefer a hand-written version.

Food Journal Example:

My Food Journal					
Date	Time	Food	Meal/ Snack	Emotion	How Hungry?
Exercise done for the week:					

There is no right or wrong way to record what you eat. You can use this chart as a guideline. Feel free to be as creative and descriptive as you like.

Wholey Cow Tips:

1. Take note of how you feel after eating grains. Look for dark circles under your eyes, skin conditions or a sluggish feeling.
2. If you have no issues with grains, you might want to experiment. Try something new and different such as quinoa or buckwheat.
3. Try adding a grain you don't normally use in to a breakfast meal for an additional serving of protein and boost of vitamins.
4. Add more good-fats to your diet, including avocados, nuts, seeds, olives, dark chocolate, coconut oil, olive oil, grape seed oil and a variety of fish.
5. Start a food journal to track your food choices, patterns and emotions.

PRINCIPLE #3

REACH FOR RAINBOW COLORS

REACH FOR RAINBOW COLORS

"Colors are the smiles of nature."
—Leigh Hunt

Eating a healthy diet is the best way to give your body the vitamins and minerals it needs. Some of the best sources of these powerful nutrients come from fruit and vegetables. These two types of whole foods help nourish your body. Moreover, they contain powerful antioxidants that help fight free radicals. Sadly, many people do not eat enough of them, especially vegetables.

Perhaps you grew up with your mother telling you to eat your vegetables, but did you listen to her wisdom? Most mothers know vegetables are important and needed for growth. They are critical for both development and well-being.

DID YOU KNOW?

Vegetables contain vital nutrients your body needs and you can't get them from other food sources or just vitamins.

That is why it is important to eat your vegetables and plenty of them. Instead of asking, "Where's the beef?" you should be asking, "Where are the beets?" or this vegetable or that vegetable. Let's face it, health problems and obesity weren't created by eating too many vegetables.

When I was diagnosed with an iron deficiency, whole foods became extremely important to me. I chose to focus on eating more vegetables, especially greens, as I wasn't necessarily eating them at every meal. Unfortunately, this is common for a large amount of people.

The good news is you can make better choices when it comes to your diet. When sitting down for a meal, make sure you reach for plenty of colorful foods. Our eyes are naturally drawn to bright colors, so adding them to your plate should be effortless. Choose carrots, asparagus, tomatoes, peppers, beets, eggplant, yellow squash or sweet corn to add a burst of color.

Here's a list that breaks down a few vegetable nutrients by color:

Rainbow Colored Vegetables

Red:
Red vegetables typically contain nutrients good for your heart and eyes. They are a good source of vitamins A and C.

Yellow:
Yellow vegetables are sure to brighten any plate. Yellow peppers contain vitamin C. Yellow sweet corn and yellow summer squash are rich in the antioxidant, lutein and zeaxanthin, and help fight free radicals to protect your eyes.

Green:
Green vegetables are loaded with a variety of nutrients. Greens, especially the dark, leafy varieties such as kale and spinach, contain potassium, iron and vitamin A. Green peppers and broccoli are excellent sources of vitamin C. Green vegetables come in a variety of different shades, so you won't get bored in the selection process.

Orange:
Orange colored vegetables are a great source of vitamin A, which helps promote good vision and healthy teeth. Think carrots, pumpkin, squash and sweet potatoes when choosing orange vegetables. Don't be shy adding orange bell peppers to your salad or your stir fry. They provide a healthy dose of vitamin C.

Purple:
Purple colored vegetables aren't as plentiful as some other colored vegetables. There are a few purple colored vegetables that are fairly common though, including eggplant, purple potatoes and purple cabbage. Both eggplant and purple potatoes contain antioxidants to help improve memory. Make sure you leave the peel on these vegetables to help enhance their antioxidant benefits.[19]

Add More Greens to Your Diet

Most people are familiar with going green, which is good for the environment. Going green is also good for your health. Greens are rich in calcium, magnesium, phosphorus, zinc, and the vitamins A, C, E and K.

What are greens?

Greens:
Dark, leafy vegetables that grow above the ground. Greens contain a host of vitamins and nutrients your body thrives upon.

Some popular greens include:

- Spinach
- Kale
- Collards
- Swiss Chard
- Cabbage
- Arugula
- Romaine lettuce
- Radicchio

Greens provide a host of benefits including improved circulation, blood purification, improved liver and kidney function, a strengthened immune system and more. Greens, conversely, are the most common missing food for many people today. While some people may enjoy a salad for lunch or dinner, not everyone is keen on greens. Greens provide many vitamins you can't get in other ways. In order to get their healthful benefits, you should include them at every meal. Think of greens as a ground covering for your plate. Adding greens to your diet does not have to be complicated. It can be as easy as adding a handful or two to a stir fry, chow mein or spaghetti. There are many possibilities.

Add More Vegetables to Your Daily Eating Routine

Have you ever noticed you feel different when you eat whole foods versus processed foods? Whole foods contain the nutrients your body was made to thrive upon, so you naturally feel better. Vegetables are loaded with these feel-good nutrients, so you can't go wrong by eating more. Where can you add more to your diet? Maybe lunch or dinner? Perhaps you could have them as an afternoon snack?

The obvious place to add more vegetables in my diet was at breakfast. This was the one meal I rarely included them. I experimented with adding spinach, onions, mushrooms and tomatoes to my eggs, hash browns and other breakfast foods. In addition, I started adding spinach, kale and a variety of other healthful items to my breakfast smoothies.

Smoothies can be fun to make, as there are plenty of options. Start by selecting a few vegetables to increase your nutrient intake. Play around and see what appeals to your tastes. For an added boost of energy, try adding some super foods like coconut oil, maca powder, cacao nibs or chia seeds. To get your morning dose of protein, you can add protein powder, peanut butter, nuts or seeds.

> **What are Super Foods?**
>
> **Super Foods:**
> Foods considered nutrient dense that are especially beneficial to the body. Eating super foods helps to promote overall health and well-being.[20]

Avocados are another nutritious item you can add to your smoothie. Avocados are rich in vitamin A and potassium and contain healthy fat and fiber your body craves. Some nutrition experts rank them as one of the top five healthiest foods on the planet. Avocados are actually considered a fruit, but I always think of them as a vegetable. It doesn't really matter how they are classified—just remember they are healthy and good for you.

Making green juice is another way you can add more vegetables to your diet. Green juice provides a quick energy boost and plenty of nutrients. Try juicing spinach, kale, cucumbers, celery, other greens, or carrots. I was never a fan of vegetable juice, but after experimenting a little, the taste grew on me. It didn't take long to notice a difference in my energy level and my iron naturally began to climb. As an added bonus, I became less prone to getting sick.

Incorporate More Sweet Vegetables

Many people have a sweet tooth, but grabbing a donut, cookie or sugar-filled drink is not the best way to curb a sweet craving. There are plenty of healthful choices you can make, such as adding sweet vegetables to your diet. Sweet vegetables are good for you and can help provide a boost of nutrients to your daily intake. Sweet vegetables can help satisfy cravings for other sweets too.

Make sure you snack on plenty of crunchy vegetables including carrots, bell peppers, snap peas, beets, broccoli, celery and others.

Fruits—Nature's Candy

Another way to increase your daily intake of vitamins and fiber is to add fruit to your diet. Fruit contains plenty of natural sugars, but unlike cake, ice cream or donuts, fruit has plenty of health benefits. Fruit digests slower than most processed foods and triggers satiety hormones to help prevent over eating. What's more, fruit contains essential vitamins, flavonoids and antioxidants. Strive to eat 1 to 2 servings of fruit per day.

Fruit comes in a variety of colors, shapes and sizes. Consumers naturally reach for apples, oranges and bananas because of their bright colors. Berries are another popular choice for consumers and are loaded with phytochemicals, antioxidants and minerals. Berries like blueberries, raspberries and strawberries are considered super foods since they are nutrient-rich and promote well-being. Berries help fight inflammation, strengthen the immune system and help fight cancer. Many people love the sweet taste of berries and enjoy them as a snack. You can also add them to yogurt, smoothies or make a pie with them. Grapes are another fruit loaded with phytochemicals and antioxidants and help protect your body from cancer and other disease. Plus—they help prevent heart disease. Choose red, purple and blue varieties. Grapes are great for snacking and make a nutritious dessert.

Wholey Cow Tips:

1. Fill your plate with brightly colored vegetables.
2. Cover a large portion of your plate with greens (think grass-cover for your plate).
3. Make sure you eat vegetables at every meal. Snack on crunchy vegetables such as carrots, broccoli, celery, bell peppers or asparagus.
4. Add more sweet vegetables to your diet such as carrots or sugar snap peas. They are good for you and may help satisfy your sweet craving.
5. Add greens to smoothies, eggs, potatoes or side dishes, such as rice or quinoa.
6. Experiment with green juice. It is a great way to add vegetables in your diet, as well as more nutrients.
7. Eat a variety of fruits to boost your fiber intake.
8. Focus on eating 1-2 servings of fruit per day.
9. Choose berries such as blueberries, raspberries and strawberries, as well as grapes, to help get a healthy dose of phytochemicals and antioxidants.

PRINCIPLE #4

LESS IS MORE!

Less Is More!

"Simplicity is the ultimate sophistication."
—Leonardo da Vinci

Sugar Shock!

Oh—sugar! How sweet it is! Delicious, tempting, tantalizing and deadly! Yes—deadly! Most people love sugar, have been deceived by its sweet flavor and addictive properties, and have become accustomed to it in just about everything. Many nutrition experts, however, believe sugar is a toxin and the cause of many diseases.

DID YOU KNOW?

According to some experts, sugar is to blame for obesity, type 2 diabetes, heart disease, hypertension and cancer.[21]

Those are some harsh facts and something you might want to consider the next time you want to bite into a chocolate chip cookie.

Most people associate sugar with sweets. Yet sugar is included in almost everything processed today. Sugar is masked under dozens of different names, making it hard to identify. Sugar can be found in the form of high fructose corn syrup, maltose, molasses, dextrin, fructose, dextrose, dextran, barley malt, evaporated can juice, rice syrup, sucrose and the list goes on. It's easy to see how consumers are confused and end up eating so much of it.

A lot of people can't imagine removing sugar entirely from their diet. You can definitely make an effort to bring your sugar consumption down, though. I recently saw an interesting interview with a well-known doctor and author in the field of health and nutrition, who described sugar as a recreational drug, which is ok to eat occasionally.[22] I thought this was kind of funny, although very true. The analogy is similar to that of consuming alcohol. You can't just eat sugar all day long and not expect it to have some sort of effect. It is hard on your body. This is a big problem and is part of what is feeding the obesity epidemic.

Processed Food

Grocery stores today are packed with processed foods and consumers are all too familiar with them. Have you ever stopped to consider how processed foods came about and why many are considered unhealthy?

What is a processed food?

Processed Food:
Any food altered from its natural state.

Some common processed foods include microwave popcorn, chips, crackers, macaroni and cheese, pizza, bread, cereal, soup, cheese, meat products, condiments and more.

Processed foods have received a bad rap over the years, yet a number of them aren't bad. A variety of processed foods are minimally processed— think bagged vegetables, salads, nuts and seeds. These products simply contain a few ingredients, so are considered safe and wholesome.

Heavily processed foods, on the other hand, are the ones you should avoid. These products typically contain large amounts of trans-fats, sodium, sugar and high fructose corn syrup. Chemicals, artificial ingredients and preservatives are also found in a lot of these products. Many of them are masked with hard-to-pronounce names, making them difficult to identify.

Processed foods have been around since before the turn of the century. As trans-fats were introduced in the early 1900s, more and more processed foods began to trickle in to the food supply and have been growing since.[23] Processed foods gained popularity in the 80s as more artificial sweeteners became available. The real explosion of processed foods took place in the 90s when the low-fat craze came about. Today you can find processed foods in grocery stores, gas stations, office supply stores, big-box stores and more.

Processed foods aren't the healthiest choice. Consumers, nonetheless continue to buy them because they are convenient to make, eat and buy. Many processed foods are less expensive than whole foods, making them affordable to many. Additionally, there are thousands of choices, making them both appealing and compelling. When buying processed foods, shoot for products containing five ingredients or less. Take your time when grocery shopping to ensure you find the best choices.

Sugar-Filled Drinks

When it comes to weight gain, sugar-filled drinks are part of the problem for many individuals. Did you know there are a whopping 39 grams of sugar in a can of coke? Yes, 39![24] This is equivalent to about 9-1/2 teaspoons! Can you imagine consciously adding such a large amount of sugar to your coffee or tea? Most people who drink soda pop don't realize they are ingesting so much sugar. Those who purchase 20 oz. bottles or super-sized drinks consume even more sugar.

To avoid all the sugar in regular soda pop, some people opt for diet soda pop. The truth is diet soda pop is not good for you either. Diet soda pop is loaded with chemicals your body doesn't necessarily know how to process. Artificial sweeteners such as aspartame, saccharin and sucralose are used to sweeten diet soda pops and are sweeter than sugar. Studies show that when these sweeteners are consumed over time, individuals crave more sweets. If you want to avoid both the sugar and chemicals, it is best to steer clear of soda pop in general. If you like the fizz of soda pop, why not try sparkling water as an alternative? Sparkling water provides the carbonation bubbles like soda pop and comes in a variety of flavors.

Soda pop is not the only problem when it comes to sugar-filled drinks and weight gain. Many coffee drinks are loaded with sugar. People have enjoyed coffee for years, but with the rising popularity of coffee shops, coffee has taken on a whole new twist. Coffee shops are trendy and offer consumers a variety of specialty drink choices. Sorry to say, most specialty drinks are loaded with sugar. Many consumers don't think about what is in their caramel latte or café mocha and focus instead on the taste.

Did you know a 12 oz. caramel frappuccino non-fat blended coffee from Starbucks has a whopping 47 grams of sugar! A 16 oz. version of the same drink has 66 grams![25] Talk about a quick sugar high! It is easy to see how people gain weight when consuming these drinks on a consistent basis.

Coffee shops most likely won't eliminate sugar from their products any time soon. You can make healthier drink choices when you visit, however. Why not purchase a medium roast coffee and add your own cream and sugar? You can use stevia, honey or another alternate to cut back on your sugar consumption. Your taste-buds will adjust to the taste and I guarantee you will be happier with your choice.

I am not a coffee drinker, yet I do enjoy tea. A number of years ago, I got hooked on drinking chai tea from a local coffee shop. I loved the taste, but noticed over a period of time, I put on a few pounds. I quickly decided it was time to make my own, healthier version. Now I use stevia to sweeten my tea and prefer the taste over sugar. If you like tea, you may want to try an unsweetened version or herbal variety. Green tea is always a good choice, as it is loaded with antioxidants.

Wholey Cow Tips:

1. Try alternative natural sweeteners such as honey, maple syrup or agave in place of sugar to sweeten your tea or oatmeal.
2. Avoid food products that contain a lot of sugar or have sugar listed as one of the first ingredients on the label.
3. Avoid foods with aspartame, sucralose and saccharin. These chemical-based sweeteners have been shown to cause serious side effects.
4. Try stevia as an alternate sweetener to sugar. It is plant-derived and sweeter than sugar, so use this sweetener sparingly. Look for organic, good quality stevia, as some forms of stevia are altered and have additional ingredients to give them a longer shelf life.
5. Look for recipes using coconut or dried fruits such as dates, raisins, currants, prunes or cherries instead of sugar.
6. Try cutting down on soda pop, or better yet, remove it altogether from your diet.

PRINCIPLE #5

QUALITY VS. QUANTITY—
MAKE CONSCIOUS CHOICES

QUALITY VS. QUANTITY— MAKE CONSCIOUS CHOICES

"Quality is never an accident. It is always the result of intelligent effort."
—John Ruskin

From Super-Size to Super-Wise

Isn't it strange how large portions of food have become common place in our society, over the years? From meat, French fries, soda pop and more, everything seems to be bigger, including the plates. It's not surprising given the fact that the media often leads us astray. We are constantly bombarded with messages saying, "You need more!" From the classic 1984 Wendy's commercial titled, "Where's the beef?" to the 90s McDonald's "Super Size It" campaign, it is no wonder we all got confused!

Other restaurants soon followed the Super Size trend. It didn't take long to figure out the serve more and charge more concept. Many consumers bought into this trend and felt it was a good value. When you eat out, you typically eat more.

DID YOU KNOW?

People who eat out consume 200 calories or more than at home. That adds up and can result in up to 20 pounds of extra weight in a year.[26]

That is a lot of extra weight, especially if you multiply it over a few years. So much for Super-Sizing your meals! You can see this concept back fired.

To avoid overeating when going out, you can make conscious choices to eat less and choose healthier items. For example, you could split a meal with your spouse, significant other or friend. Ask for an extra plate or have the restaurant divide the portions of food. If you are eating alone, split the meal in half before you start eating. Ask your server for a box to bring the other half home to eat for another meal. Consider asking the server if the restaurant offers smaller portions or lunch sizes. Another option is to order off the appetizer menu, as a number of appetizers may work for a meal.

Another way to make conscious choices to eat healthier is to make substitutions for unhealthy items such as fries and chips. Many restaurants offer side salads, steamed vegetables, fruit and more. Certain restaurants might offer a "healthy" or "light" section on their menu. You may find a healthier item in this section and leave the restaurant feeling better than if you ordered a standard burger and fries.

Make Smarter Choices

A lot of people have got in the habit of eating out several times a week or more. A healthier choice is to make more home cooked meals. Eating at home allows you to choose healthier ingredients and serve more properly proportioned meals.

Meal-prep starts with a list of wholesome ingredients. Look for more whole foods when you are out shopping. The best place to find them is the perimeter of the grocery store. The produce section, meat department, dairy and bakery are all located on the outside edges of the store. Shopping this way is much easier and less stressful. Sometimes I don't even venture to other isles, unless I need something specific like a spice, tea or a condiment.

Look for good quality fruits and vegetables when out shopping, if possible. Organic produce is your best bet, as it is grown without the use of artificial chemicals. If you are price conscious, feel free to go with conventional produce. Make sure to thoroughly wash the fruit and vegetables you buy to remove any residue or wax build up.

If you are concerned about pesticides and produce, you might want to take a look at the website for the Environmental Working Group, which provides a Shopper's Guide to Pesticides in Produce list you can easily download.[27] Take the list with you when you shop to easily determine which produce is heavily sprayed.

What is the Dirty Dozen?

Dirty Dozen:

12 of the most heavily sprayed produce available.

1. Strawberries
2. Spinach
3. Nectarines
4. Apples
5. Peaches
6. Pears
7. Cherries
8. Grapes
9. Celery
10. Tomatoes
11. Sweet Bell Peppers
12. Potatoes

Plus:

13. Hot Peppers

What is the Clean 15?

Clean 15:

A list of the least likely produce to be sprayed and contaminated with pesticides. You should feel comfortable buying these conventional items, unless you prefer buying organic produce.

1. Sweet Corn
2. Avocados
3. Pineapples
4. Cabbage
5. Onions
6. Sweet Peas
7. Papayas
8. Asparagus
9. Mangos
10. Eggplant
11. Honeydew
12. Kiwi
13. Cantaloupe
14. Cauliflower
15. Grapefruit[28]

Note: The EWG updates this periodically. This is the 2017 list.

Buy Local

Another way to make conscious choices when buying produce is to buy local. Some grocery stores offer locally grown produce during the growing season from farmers in their area. Look for fresh sweet corn, tomatoes, cucumbers, potatoes and green beans.

If you can't find the fresh produce you want at your local grocery store, try looking for a farmers market nearby. Farmers markets offer local farmers, artists and crafters a way to sell their products directly to the public. Farmers markets typically offer a retail setting of booths and tables staffed by various vendors and farmers. Farmers generally offer an array of seasonal produce including peppers, corn, asparagus, tomatoes, pumpkins, squash, apples, strawberries and more. Some farmers sell meat, eggs and honey. Other items such as flowers and wild rice may be available from certain vendors. Other prepared items such as bread, pickles, baked goods, canned pickles and crafts may be available, as well. It all depends on what is on hand in your region. If you haven't visited a farmers market before, you might want to give one a try. Farmers markets can be found in cities across the country. Farmers markets offer fresh food and provide a good way to support your local farmer and community.

Join a Community Supported Agriculture (CSA) Group

Another way to buy locally grown food in your region is to join a CSA group.

What is a Community Supported Agriculture Group?

Community Supported Agriculture (CSA) Group:
CSA groups are made up of farmers in a particular area who work directly with consumers to buy their crops. These farmers typically offer a number of "crop shares" to people in their community before the season begins.[29]

Most CSA farmers offer a membership program, where you pay a fee upfront. During the growing season, you typically receive a box of fresh produce weekly.

CSAs benefit both the farmer and the consumer. They work well for large families, day cares and individuals who like to can vegetables, as they provide substantial quantities of produce. If you are single or have a smaller family, contact your local CSA for more information. They should be able to answer questions regarding membership pricing and weekly produce quantities.

Wholey Cow Tips:

1. When eating out, order only one entrée and share it with another person, when possible.
2. Split the meal in half before you start eating. Eat only one half of the meal and box the other to bring home and eat for another meal.
3. Ask the restaurant if they serve smaller portions or lunch sizes of an item (e.g. order a half salad or a cup of soup instead of a bowl).
4. Order a salad or a vegetable in place of a potato or rice and eat it before the main entrée to fill up more on greens or vegetables before the protein portion of the meal.
5. If the restaurant has a "light" or "healthy" section, place your order from there.
6. Make more meals at home.
7. Pay attention to the Dirty Dozen and Clean 15. You can get a copy of the guide from the Environmental Working Group at: https://www.ewg.org/foodnews/.
8. Buy local or organic if possible. To find a CSA near you or investigate joining a CSA in your area, check out Local Harvest at: http://www.localharvest.org/csa/

BEYOND FOOD

PRINCIPLE #6

ASK WHAT'S MISSING

Ask What's Missing

"Let us read, and let us dance - these two amusements will never do harm to the world."
—Voltaire

Recipe for Renewal

Eating terrible food, not getting enough rest and working too many hours can put a strain on your body and mind. This often leads to stress and other symptoms such as weight gain, mood swings, headaches and tension. Over time, more severe symptoms may occur and eventually disease can develop. Sadly, the majority of doctors fail to look at your overall health and instead treat the symptoms with drugs. Unfortunately, this type of doctoring works more like a Band-Aid—it covers the problem, yet does not necessarily find a solution to the underlying cause.

There is a different theory out there, however, on how to restore health. This perspective involves two types of foods that feed us—primary foods and secondary foods. Primary foods include relationships, physical activity, career and spirituality. These foods feed you at a much deeper level—your soul—and can satisfy your hunger for life. Secondary foods are the foods you take into our body.[30] Even though it is important to eat plenty of healthy foods, it is critical you get a healthy dose of primary foods. They are the foundation of well-being. When you neglect your body, you also hurt the ones you love.

For optimal health, consider focusing on feeding your primary foods. Exercising, reading, spending quality time with others, feeding your spirit and working is a great recipe for renewal in life.[31]

Social Satiety

Relationships play a big part in our day-to-day lives and can have a significant role in how you feel. Healthy relationships with family, friends, co-workers and neighbors can help you feel grounded. Besides this, significant relationships can make you feel needed by others and provide a sense of community. Having a relationship with a spouse or significant other can provide intimacy and someone to share personal experiences with. Whether you are married single or dating, everyone needs relationships of some sort to feel connected.

People who don't have enough relationships in their life may feel lost and lonely. Feelings of emptiness can arise when you don't have enough close friends, or are away from family. Physical symptoms may appear in the body if you don't have enough connections with other humans. Your body may be crying out for human touch and emotional sharing. When you love someone, have interactions with another and place importance on others, you feel naturally better overall.

If you lack significant relationships in your life, it is important to establish more. For example, if you have a job where you don't have a lot of contact with people or are a stay at home mom, make sure you explore opportunities to meet others. Maybe you could join a church group, a mom's group, a bowling league, health club, golf league or a tennis team? Volunteering is another option. Make sure you find something that interests you and sign up. If you like to read, why not join a book club? Most book clubs meet regularly. Look for a club that covers topics and books you enjoy. The possibilities are endless. The important thing is to figure out what you like and find others with similar interests. Relationships will naturally follow.

Appetizing Activities

Taking care of your body includes not only eating the right foods, but also activity and exercise. Your body was meant to move and not be sedentary. There are a variety of ways to add exercise and physical activity to your life. Whether you like to walk, bike, run, lift weights, ski, play tennis, golf, play basketball or do yoga, it is important to stay active.

Exercise can be fun and exhilarating and can make you feel more alive physically. Fitting exercise in your day, however, can sometimes be challenging. Most people live busy lives, so exercise needs to be a priority. Make sure you schedule time to exercise in your day. If you don't like going to the gym and find yourself making excuses not to go, you might need to change your mind-set about exercise. Try not to get caught up on what you don't like and focus instead on finding an activity you enjoy. There are plenty of activities you can do.

This reminds me of an incident that happened to me recently. I happened to watch Bruce Springstein's, Dancing In The Dark YouTube video when some visitors were over. I hadn't seen the video in a long time and it sure brought back some good memories from college life. Those were fun, care-free times. Although I wouldn't want to go back, it made me think about growing up and all of the fun things I enjoyed—like dancing. I am not sure why I stopped. This happens with many people—as you age, it is easy to get wrapped up in your job, your family, your problems and daily chores, and you lose your spark over time. It is easy to see how you might get "tired and bored with yourself."

So why does this happen and how can you re-ignite your fire? Many people tax their body by eating terrible food, not getting enough rest and working too many hours. These behaviors can lead to symptoms of stress, anxiety, weight gain and a multitude of other disorders.

This reminds me of another scenario with plants. Wise gardeners know to dig up the root system of a plant when the leaves start to look sick. In order for the leaves to be healthy, the roots need to be strong.[32] As with plants, we need to look at the root cause for health. Sadly, our current medical system is focused on symptoms rather than the cause of them and many people end up just popping pills. You may merely be lacking some primary food, like exercise, to remedy your problems. Why not take the time to find out what activity you really like as an alternative? It doesn't have to be some popular exercise either. What activities did you enjoy as a child? Why not give one a try again and see how it makes you feel?

DID YOU KNOW?

Finding an exercise you enjoy may be as easy as looking back at your childhood.

I personally love to exercise and have always incorporated a variety of activities into my routine. I walk daily and enjoy biking, yoga, weight training and water skiing. I also include some non-traditional activities in my exercise regimen now and again. You can find me hula hooping, jumping on a trampoline and swinging. I just love these activities. They remind me of my childhood and raising my children. Additionally, they make me smile and laugh, so why not? Remember, there is no age limit on having fun and we are all kids at heart. So go ahead and swing, jump, skip or dance. Try whatever activity gets you going and then get going on it.

Wonderful Work

Although there are a number of people who claim to have the perfect job, it unrealistic to think one exists for everyone. If you love what you do, that is great. If you are like most people, you probably like the majority of your tasks, but not necessarily everything. This is normal.

Working takes up a large part of the day, so it is important to have tasks you enjoy. Most people can find fulfillment in their work if they have enough pleasing responsibilities.

If you don't have enough tasks you enjoy and are not fulfilled, you may want to consider finding another job. If a new job isn't the right answer, maybe you can find a hobby or another activity you are fond of to fill in some gaps. Remember, life is too short to spend it being unhappy so go out and search for something meaningful to you.

Soul Food

Religion plays an integral part in the lives of many and provides an important system of beliefs. Many people like going to church and enjoy the faith, worship and community it offers. There are others, however, who prefer less formality and structure. Whether you are religious or more spiritual, everyone needs time alone to think, meditate and reflect. Having a spiritual practice is a great way to connect to God and your higher-self. The time you spend alone each day can help clear your mind and give you time to think. It can also provide a sense of balance in your life. Silent time can be used for reflecting, praying or just thinking good, positive thoughts. Silence allows us time to re-connect with ourselves and helps bring peace and contentment.

Meditation can be a form of spirituality. Meditation can help you to re-connect to yourself and promotes a sense of well-being. Despite the fact that mediation is good for you, many people have a difficult time with it. It is hard to still the mind and sit silently focusing on the present moment, and it takes a great deal of practice. If you are a beginner, make sure you sit in stillness for only a few minutes at a time and build from there. If your mind starts to wander, just start again and keep practicing. Over time, you will be able to sit silently longer. Even meditating for several minutes is beneficial for both your mind and body.

Some people prefer other meditative practices such as Yoga and Tai Chi to still the mind. Others may choose to practice a meditative walk or swim.

I personally prefer a morning meditative walk, as it fills me with a sense of peace and calm. Sometimes I practice certain mantras as I walk or say some prayers. Other times I listen to something inspirational. I always try to keep my thoughts simple and enjoy the sunshine on my face and the chirping of the birds. My morning walks help keep me balanced and positive.

How about you? Are you spending time alone or incorporating a spiritual or meditative practice? If not, I suggest you give it try. It won't take long for you to see the benefits. Many people who have a spiritual or meditative practice feel a little off when they miss a day. It is funny how our body and mind adapt and longs for this time of renewal.

Savoring Self-Care

Many people are good at taking care of others, but when it comes to taking care of themselves, it can be another story. This is especially true for women. Women tend to be the caregivers of the family and frequently put the needs of others in front of their own. This is unfortunate, as in order to take good care of others, you need time to renew your own body and mind. How can you possibly take care of others if you are running yourself ragged? Some people have a hard time understanding this concept, yet we all need self-care to renew our energy.

There are a quite a number of ways to practice self-care. It can be as simple as choosing something you like doing, such as going to a movie, concert, or shopping. Getting a massage can have a positive effect on your body, too. It relaxes your muscles and helps to detoxify your body. Taking a nap is another way to rejuvenate your body and can give you a boost of energy for the rest of the day.

Having a manicure, pedicure or getting your hair done is another way to treat yourself. These services can help you escape the stresses of daily living. They can boost self-esteem to boot, by making you feel better about your appearance. I used to have a hard time pampering myself. Although I get my hair done regularly, having a massage or pedicure was something I did only on occasion. This is common for many of us. As I learned how important self-care is for my mind and body, I changed my thoughts and now schedule a massage monthly and look forward to it.

Reading is another way to have some time alone and escape. If you enjoy reading, take at least 10 minutes a day to read a good book, magazine or journal. When you are reading and learning, you are improving yourself and naturally feel happier.

Another way to practice self-care is to take a vacation. We all need time to get away from our daily routines and work life. Why not schedule a vacation to rest, relax and rejuvenate your body? If you like the sun and beach, look for a warm destination. If you like adventure, why not plan a trip involving exploration, hiking, biking or site-seeing? There are many possibilities. If you can't afford to get away by plane or train, try planning a vacation nearby. Why not schedule some fun activities you wouldn't normally do? Check with your local library, Chamber of Commerce or do a Google search to find fun things to do in your area. You might be surprised by how many ideas you find. It doesn't matter what you do on your vacation. The important thing is to get away and out of your regular routine.

Take a few minutes and jot down some things you can try to rejuvenate your mind, body and spirit.

Wholey Cow Self-Care Ideas:

1. _____
2. _____
3. _____
4. _____
5. _____
6. _____
7. _____
8. _____
9. _____
10. _____

Wholey Cow Tips:

1. Explore avenues to create fulfilling relationships. You can join a church group, bowling league, health club, golf league or tennis team.
2. Take some time to exercise each day. If you haven't found an exercise you like, think back to your childhood to help remember some things you enjoyed doing.
3. Develop a spiritual practice if you don't have one. Take some time each day to be alone.
4. Incorporate more self-care in your life. Take time to read, relax and pamper yourself.

WHOLE YOU!

PRINCIPLE #7

TAKE CHARGE

TAKE CHARGE

"Action is the foundational key to all success."
—Pablo Picasso

Choose To Make a Difference

Now that you are familiar with some basic principles for healthy eating and living, it is time to take charge. How can you make conscious choices about what you eat and where should you begin? A good place to start is with your refrigerator and pantry. The kitchen is the heart of the home and should be a place of nourishment. To avoid temptation, try and remove all sugary-snacks and highly processed foods that can be addicting and may pack on the pounds. Stock up on real foods mentioned in the *In the Beginning* section including vegetables, fruit, grains, spices, nuts, seeds and meat (fish, chicken and beef).

If you are not ready to give up all of your favorites, don't worry. No one is perfect. When it comes to eating healthy, you might want to follow the 80/20 rule. Try to eat whole foods, including lots of vegetables and protein, at least 80% of the time. This way of eating gives you a little lee-way so you can still have the slice of the pizza you love from time to time. If you eat healthy during the week, you can feel comfortable going to a restaurant over the weekend with friends and maybe having a few fries with your entrée.

DID YOU KNOW?
Following an 80/20 diet can give you a
healthy mindset for eating.

If you have more will power than most, try following the 90/10 rule. This way of eating is even healthier and still gives you the opportunity to indulge from time to time.

Over Haul Your Diet

If you are ready to make a life-style change by incorporating wholesome eating habits, there are a few simple things you can do to get started. If you follow them, you will be on your way to healthy eating and living.

Eat Breakfast

Breakfast is thought to be the most important meal of the day, according to many nutrition experts. After a long night's sleep, eating breakfast gets the body going and gives you energy for the day ahead. It is ironic that breakfast is the most skipped meal. Both children and adults are guilty of missing this important meal. Many people feel rushed in the morning and don't necessarily allow enough time to grab something to eat before heading out the door. Do yourself a favor and take a little time to eat something healthy. Breakfast doesn't have to be hard to make or complicated. Try mixing a few healthful ingredients together to make a smoothie. Maybe try a banana, handful of spinach and some protein powder. Use whatever fruits and vegetables you like. There are many possibilities. If you are in a rush, grab a banana and yogurt. If you have a little extra time, make yourself some eggs. Try adding in some healthy vegetables and maybe some leftover chicken or ham. Again, you have many options. The point is to eat something healthy, preferably with protein and vegetables.

Pre-Plan Meals

When it comes to cooking, doing a little pre-planning can make your life and meals easier. Make a list of meals you would like to make. If you want to try something new, find some healthy recipes you would like to try. Use one of your favorite cookbooks, some favorite recipe cards or search Pinterest.

If you have kids, make sure you get them involved in the process. Start by making a list of several meals you would like to make. Make a grocery list of the items you don't have on hand and need to purchase. Take the kids or other family members to the grocery store and have them help pick out any items needed. Once you have your groceries, you can prepare several items ahead to make things easier for the week. You can chop vegetables in advance for salads, snacking and stir-fries. Store them in glass containers, so they are easily visible and ready "to go." If you plan to make a dish with chicken, why not cook a few extra chicken breasts? This way, you will have them on hand for salads, chicken fajitas or another meal. Pre-planning saves time, gives you a set plan of meals and allows you to eat healthier. What's more, you will be less likely to visit that local restaurant for a greasy burger and fries.

Replace Bad Oils with Good Oils

Calories are often hidden in unhealthy oils such as corn oil, soybean oil, sunflower oil and others. Try replacing some of these unhealthy oils with olive oil or coconut oil. These oils are anti-inflammatory and contain healthy antioxidants. Make sure you use them when cooking and baking.

Replace Snack Foods with Nuts and Seeds

Processed foods, including crackers and chips, are often loaded with chemicals and preservatives. Although they may taste good, many have addicting properties that keep you eating and wanting more. Try replacing some of these snack foods with nuts and seeds. Nuts and seeds contain good fats your body craves. They also contain protein and fiber, as well as a variety of vitamins and minerals your body needs. If you are looking for something crunchy to eat, snack on almonds, cashews, macadamia nuts, walnuts, pecans and sunflower seeds. Nuts and seeds fill you up and give you extended energy for the day. Enjoy 1 to 2 handfuls of these healthful whole foods.

Watch Out For Condiments

While many people love condiments, many are loaded with sugar and chemicals. Ketchup and mustard seem to go hand in hand with a burger and fries, but when is the last time you looked at the ingredient list? Many people slather on the ketchup, not knowing they are consuming a large dose of sugar. Ketchup is loaded with high fructose corn syrup, which essentially is sugar and is horrible for your body. Other condiments, including sauces and dressings, are also loaded with sugars and preservatives. Make sure you read the labels to identify unhealthy ingredients and hidden sugar. When choosing condiments, be selective and use them sparingly.

Make Your Own Dressings

Many dressings contain sugar and other chemicals. If you like eating salad, you might want to consider making your own dressing. Many people like vinegar and oil, but there are many other options. You can make a healthy dressing using olive oil, lemon and your favorite herbs. You can do an online search, or check out Pinterest.com, for a variety of healthy dressing choices. If you are eating out, ask for your salad dressing on the side. This way you can control the amount of dressing you put on your salad. Some restaurants offer healthier dressing selections. Make sure you ask in advance what your options are.

Look For Healthy Food Products

If you are looking to overhaul your diet, look for healthy food products. Remember, the fewer ingredients the better. If you are not ready to give up all your snack items, make sure you read the ingredient list. Some items are definitely better than others. For example, you would be better off choosing a bag of Tostitos over a bag of Doritos chips. Tostitos contain three ingredients, whereas Doritos contain many more ingredients. A much better option, of course, is to fill your pantry and refrigerator with more whole food snacks.

Eat More Good Fat

Although low-fat foods are popular, they aren't all healthy. Fat plays a big part in how a food tastes and low-fat foods often have added sugar or other chemicals to make them taste better. Opt instead for healthy fats found in an assortment of whole foods. Start buying more avocados, nuts, seeds, olives, coconut oil, olive oil, dark chocolate and a variety of fish for a healthy dose of fat.

Garden

Even though not everyone has the space to start a garden, more and more consumers like the idea of growing their own food. Gardening provides a great way to have fresh vegetables on hand. Additionally, it provides an opportunity to freeze and can fresh fruits and vegetables for later use, which is especially nice in the winter months. If you don't have room for a garden, there are still a number of ways you can grow fresh vegetables. If you have a patio or deck, why not buy a potted tomato or pepper plant? You can also grow herbs or other small plants on a window ledge. Community gardens provide another way to take up gardening. Some cities have designated spots to plant. If you live near one, why not sign up for a plot or rent some space to harvest your own vegetables? A number of schools have garden plots available as well. If you happen to live by one, you might be able to volunteer a little time or encourage your children to participate.

Create A Compost for Fertilizer

If you have a garden, why not start a compost pile if you have the room?

What is compost?

Compost:
Decomposed organic material that is used for natural fertilizer.

Starting a compost pile is easy and provides a natural way to fertilize your garden. You can dump coffee grounds, banana peels, potato peels, grass clippings, leaves and more. Why not recycle some of your garbage and make your garden flourish at the same time? Composts provide a great way to avoid harsh chemicals and fertilizers that are bad for the environment.

Wholey Cow Tips:

1. Remove all of the sugary-snacks and highly processed foods from your pantry and refrigerator.
2. Stock up on whole foods, including vegetables, fruit, grains, spices, nuts, seeds and meat (fish, chicken and beef).
3. Follow the 80/20 rule or 90/10 rule for eating.
4. Start a garden if you have the room. That way you can grow some of your own vegetables and can or freeze them for later use. If you don't have room for a garden, buy a potted vegetable plant or try growing some herbs in your kitchen window.
5. Start a compost pile and create a natural way to fertilize your garden.
6. Get your kids or other family members involved in planning meals. Make a list and head to the grocery store with your kids, spouse or significant other. You can assign your family individual tasks for meal preparation such as chopping vegetables, shredding cheese or measuring ingredients.

CONCLUSION

CONCLUSION

A Change Will Do You Good

Changes to our food supply and way of eating did not happen overnight. They are the result of a steady progression of change over the last fifty-plus years. Industrialization, factory farming, and innovation have brought us convenience, variety and good tasting food. Unfortunately, they have also contributed to the obesity epidemic and many health problems.

It has become clear that we all need to look at the way we eat. Many people do not like change, but change is a constant and something that is always expected over time. When it comes to our food supply and well-being, change is something that is needed and we all need to welcome.

As a consumer, you have many options and by making healthier choices, you can help drive changes in the way products are produced, farming practices, and the food sold in our grocery stores. In fact, changes are already taking place. With your help, we will continue to see more. Remember—the choices you make not only affect your health and well-being, but that of others.

I encourage you to eat well and choose more whole foods that provide life-energy and sustenance. Let's all use the wisdom of past generations to create a better, brighter, and healthful future.

WHOLEY COW QUICK REFERENCE TIPS

Principle #1 Food Is Fuel

1. Choose fruits, vegetables, whole grains, nuts, seeds and meat to get the most nutrients for your body.
2. Avoid food products containing ingredients you aren't familiar with, especially if there are a lot of them.
3. Be cautious about buying a food product with a specific packaging claim, such as fortified with extra calcium. Make sure you take the time to read all the ingredients in the product.
4. Start noticing and reading packaging labels.
5. Try to purchase food in its most simple state.

Principe #2 Know Thyself

1. Take note of how you feel after eating grains. Look for dark circles under your eyes, skin conditions or a sluggish feeling.
2. If you have no issues with grains, you might want to experiment Try something new and different such as quinoa or buckwheat.
3. Try adding a grain you don't normally use in to a breakfast meal for an additional serving of protein and boost of vitamins.
4. Add more good-fats to your diet, including avocados, nuts, seeds, olives, dark chocolate, coconut oil, olive oil, grape seed oil and a variety of fish.
5. Start a food journal to track your food choices, patterns and emotions.

Principe #3 Think Colors of the Rainbow

1. Fill your plate with brightly colored vegetables.
2. Cover a large portion of your plate with greens (think grass-cover for your plate).
3. Make sure you eat vegetables at every meal. Snack on crunchy vegetables such as carrots, broccoli, celery, bell peppers or asparagus.
4. Add more sweet vegetables to your diet such as carrots or sugar snap peas. They are good for you and may help satisfy your sweet craving.
5. Add greens to smoothies, eggs, potatoes or side dishes, such as rice or quinoa.
6. Experiment with green juice. It is a great way to add vegetables in your diet, as well as more nutrients.
7. Eat a variety of fruits to boost your fiber intake.
8. Focus on eating 1-2 servings of fruit per day.
9. Choose berries such as blueberries, raspberries and strawberries, as well as grapes, to help get a healthy dose of phytochemicals and antioxidants.

Principe #4 Less Is More

1. Try alternative natural sweeteners such as honey, maple syrup or agave in place of sugar to sweeten your tea or oatmeal.
2. Avoid food products that contain a lot of sugar or have sugar listed as one of the first ingredients on the label.
3. Avoid foods with aspartame, sucralose and saccharin. These chemical-based sweeteners have been shown to cause serious side effects.
4. Try stevia as an alternate sweetener to sugar. It is plant-derived and sweeter than sugar, so use this sweetener sparingly. Look for organic, good quality stevia as some forms of stevia are altered and have additional ingredients to give them a longer shelf life.
5. Look for recipes using coconut or dried fruits such as dates, raisins, currants, prunes or cherries instead of sugar.
6. Try cutting down on soda pop, or better yet, remove it altogether from your diet.

Principe #5 Quality vs. Quantity—Make Conscious Choices

1. When eating out, order only one entrée and share it with another person, when possible.
2. Split the meal in half before you start eating. Eat only one half of the meal and box the other to bring home and eat for another meal.
3. Ask the restaurant if they serve smaller portions or lunch sizes of an item (e.g. order a half salad or a cup of soup instead of a bowl).
4. Order a salad or a vegetable in place of a potato or rice and eat it before the main entrée to fill up more on greens or vegetables before the protein portion of the meal.
5. If the restaurant has a "light" or "healthy" section, place your order from there.
6. Make more meals at home.
7. Pay attention to the Dirty Dozen and Clean 15. You can get a copy of the guide from the Environmental Working Group at: https://www.ewg.org/foodnews/.
8. Buy local or organic if possible. To find a CSA near you or investigate joining a CSA in your area, check out Local Harvest at: http://www.localharvest.org/csa/

Principe #6 Ask What's Missing

1. Explore avenues to create fulfilling relationships. You can join a church group, bowling league, health club, golf league or tennis team.
2. Take some time to exercise each day. If you haven't found an exercise you like, think back to your childhood to help remember some things you enjoyed doing.
3. Develop a spiritual practice if you don't have one. Take some time each day to be alone.
4. Incorporate more self-care in your life. Take time to read, relax and pamper yourself.

Principe #7 Take Charge

1. Remove all of the sugary-snacks and highly processed foods from your pantry and refrigerator.
2. Stock up on whole foods, including vegetables, fruit, grains, spices, nuts, seeds and meat (fish, chicken and beef).
3. Follow the 80/20 rule or 90/10 rule for eating.
4. Start a garden if you have the room. That way you can grow some of your own vegetables and can or freeze them for later use. If you don't have room for a garden, buy a potted vegetable plant or try growing some herbs in your kitchen window.
5. Start a compost pile and create a natural way to fertilize your garden.
6. Get your kids or other family members involved in planning meals. Make a list and head to the grocery store with your kids, spouse or significant other. You can assign your family individual tasks for meal preparation such as chopping vegetables, shredding cheese or measuring ingredients.

Wholey Cow Samplers

Green Juice Blend

1 large handful spinach or kale
½ cucumber (cut in slices)
1-2 stalks celery (cut in pieces)
1 slice fresh ginger or 1 tsp. shredded
1 small banana
4 chunks fresh pineapple
1 tbsp. coconut oil
6-8 oz. water or coconut water

Add all ingredients to Ninja or Vitamix Blender or blender cup. Blend on high speed until thoroughly blended and mixed. Serve and enjoy. Recipe makes 1 serving.

Note: You can also add 1 tbsp. Apple Cider Vinegar if desired.

Spinach, Egg and Ham Breakfast Cups

6 eggs
1 cup fresh spinach leaves
1/2 cup ham (cut in pieces or cubes)
Shredded Cheese

Coat the bottom of muffin tins with olive oil. In a small bowl, crack the eggs and stir with a fork until the yolks are completely mixed with the egg white. Add the ham. Set aside. Place spinach leaves in the bottom of the greased muffin tins. Pour the egg and ham mix over the spinach. Top with the shredded cheese. Bake at 350 degrees for 15-18 minutes. Serve alone or with a slice or 2 of avocado and fruit.

Note: You can also add other vegetables such as tomatoes mushrooms or peppers.

Banana, Peanut Butter and Chocolate Smoothie

1 scoop chocolate protein powder
1 banana
1 handful spinach or kale
1 tbsp. peanut butter
1 tbsp. coconut oil
6-8 oz. water or almond or cashew milk

Add all ingredients to Ninja or Vitamix Blender or blender cup. Blend on high speed until thoroughly blended and mixed. Serve and enjoy. The recipe makes 1 serving.

Red, White and Blue Salad

3-4 cups of fresh mixed greens or spinach cleaned and torn
1/2 cup or so fresh blueberries
1/2 cup or so fresh strawberries cut in small chunks
1 oz. crumbled feta
1 tbsp Sweet Poppy Dressing

Poppy Seed Dressing
2 tbsp. honey
3 tbsp. apple cider vinegar or red wine vinegar
1/2 cup olive oil
1 tbsp. poppy seeds
Salt and pepper to taste

Directions:

Wash the greens, blueberries and strawberries. Place the greens or spinach in a large bowl. Add the blueberries and strawberries and mix together. Add the feta crumbles.

Mix together all of the ingredients for the dressing. Pour over individual salad plates.

Southwestern Salad

1 bag romaine lettuce or spring mix
2 grilled chicken breasts sliced or cut in pieces
1 small green pepper (chopped)
1 small red pepper (chopped)
1 small orange pepper (chopped)
1 small can corn
1 small can (2.25) black olives
1 ripe avocado (cubed)
1-4 oz. container feta cheese crumbles
Ranch or vinaigrette dressing

Open bag of lettuce and pour in a large bowl. Add chicken, chopped peppers, can of corn, olives, avocado and feta cheese. Toss and serve with ranch dressing.

Options: Add a small can of black beans or chopped red onion.

Balsamic Vinaigrette Dressing

1-1/2 cups balsamic vinegar
1 cup olive oil
1/2 tsp. salt
1 clove crushed garlic
1 tbsp. dijon mustard

In a small bowl, mix together all ingredients. Store the dressing in a glass jar or dressing container in refrigerator.

Chicken and Broccoli Bow Tie Pasta with Walnuts and Sage

2 chicken breasts (cut in pieces)
1 small head broccoli (break into small pieces)
1 small purple onion (diced)
1-2 garlic cloves (crushed)
1 cup chopped walnuts
3/4 pound bow tie pasta (use an organic brand if you prefer)
5 tbsp. butter
12 fresh sage leaves, coarsely chopped
2 tbsp. fresh squeezed lemon
1/2 tsp. salt
1/4 tsp. black pepper, or to taste
1 cup shredded Romano cheese

Generously coat a large skillet with olive oil. Add the chicken to the pan and brown over medium heat. Add the broccoli, onion, and garlic and sauté with the chicken until the broccoli is a little tender. Remove from heat and set aside. Spoon the mixture in to a bowl.

Place the walnuts in a large, dry non-stick pan over medium heat. Cook for 4-5 minutes, until lightly toasted. Remove the walnuts and set aside. Spoon the walnuts in a small bowl.

Cook the pasta in boiling water according to the package directions, about 10 minutes. When the pasta is almost done, melt the butter in a large skillet over medium heat. Add the sage, lemon juice, salt and pepper. Cook 1-2 minutes and then remove from heat.

Drain the pasta, reserving 1/2 cup of the cooking water, then add the pasta to the butter in skillet. Gradually add pasta water. Stir in the chicken mixture. Stir in the cheese and toss to combine. Garnish with the toasted nuts and serve.

Quinoa, Artichoke Black Bean and Tomato Bake

2 cups quinoa
4 cups chicken broth
1 can artichoke hearts
1 can black beans
1 large tomato diced
1 small can sliced black olives
1 cup sharp cheddar cheese (shredded)
Sprinkle with your favorite seasonings such as turmeric,
cayenne, Cajon, salt or pepper.

In a large pot, boil the chicken broth. Add the quinoa and turn down heat to simmer. Cook for approximately 20 minutes, stirring occasionally or follow the directions on the package for cooking time. When the quinoa is fully cooked, remove from the heat. Stir in the artichoke hearts, black beans, diced tomato and olives. Add your favorite seasonings. Grease the bottom of a 13" x 9" pan and pour the mixture in to it. Top with the shredded cheese and bake for approximately 25 minutes. Serve warm.

Warm Quinoa, Spinach, Tomato and Feta Salad

1/2 cup cooked quinoa
2 large handfuls fresh spinach
1 small red onion chopped
6-8 cherry tomatoes (halved)
1 clove garlic crushed
1/8 cup feta cheese crumbles
1/2 avocado (cut in to pieces)
Sprinkle with your favorite seasonings such as turmeric,
cayenne, Cajun, salt or pepper. You can also add soy sauce or coconut aminos.

Coat the bottom of a large frying pan with olive oil. Add the spinach, onion and garlic. Stir on medium heat, until the onion begins to brown and the spinach is slightly wilted. Sprinkle the top with your favorite seasonings. Stir in the quinoa to warm with the vegetables. Add the tomatoes and stir, until they are just warm. Spoon the salad on a plate. Add the feta cheese and avocado pieces on the top of the salad. Sprinkle with a little soy sauce or coconut aminos and serve warm.

Note: You may also add black beans, chick peas or another vegetable to the mix if you like.

Grilled Shrimp and Vegetable Medley

1 medium-sized red onion (sliced in to pieces)
1-8 oz. container large fresh mushrooms (cut into halves or thirds)
1 yellow pepper
2 medium vine-on tomatoes (sliced into pieces)
1 large handful spinach
Balsamic vinaigrette dressing
Soy sauce
Louisiana hot sauce
1-2 lb. bag large frozen shrimp
1 cup cooked Basmati rice

Add the onion, mushrooms and pepper slices to a grill pan. Cook on medium heat, until the vegetables begin to get soft. Sprinkle/baste with the balsamic vinaigrette, soy sauce and some Louisiana hot sauce and stir. When the vegetables are tender, add in the shrimp and cook until the shrimp becomes pinkish, about 10 minutes or so. Continue to baste and sprinkle with the balsamic vinaigrette, soy sauce and some Louisiana hot sauce. When the shrimp is done, add the tomatoes and spinach to warm. Baste again. Serve warm over rice.

Black Bean, Spinach and Chicken Tostados

2 chicken breasts (cut in pieces)
1/2 can black beans
1 small purple onion (chopped)
1 large handful spinach or other power greens
Cajun seasoning or other favorite seasoning
1 small avocado (cut into slices)
1 small Roma tomato (cut into slices)
Tostado shells
Shredded cheddar cheese (sprinkle to taste)
Salsa

Coat a medium size frying pan with olive oil. Add the chicken pieces and brown on low heat until cooked through. Add the onion and black beans and stir into the chicken. Add the spinach or other greens. Stir until the vegetables are cooked and warm. Add the Cajun or other seasoning and stir into the mix. Set aside when done. Place your tostado shell on a plate. Add the chicken and veg-etable mix. Top with the shredded cheese. Add avocado slices and tomato slices to garnish the top. Serve with salsa if desired.

Spinach, Brie and Artichoke Dip

1 small bag spinach
1 can artichoke hearts
1 wheel of Brie (cut in pie shaped pieces)
1-5 oz. container of Parmesan cheese
1 handful sliced cherry tomatoes
Crushed red pepper (sprinkle to taste)
Olive oil

Lightly coat a 13" x 9" baking pan with olive oil. Sprinkle the spinach over the olive oil. (You may only need a half of the bag, depending on the size.) Sprinkle the artichoke hearts on top of the spinach. Add the pie shaped pieces of Brie on top of the artichokes and spinach. Top with the Parmesan cheese. Add the sliced cherry tomatoes. Sprinkle with crushed red peppers to taste. Bake at 350 degrees for 20 minutes. Serve with garlic bread, corn chips or crackers.

Baked Salmon with Fresh Herbs and Black Olives

2-4 pieces of salmon (thawed)
1 small can (2.25 oz.) black olives (sliced)
Fresh parsley (chopped) (2-3 stems)
2-4 fresh basil leaves (chopped)
2-3 fresh rosemary stems (chopped)
2 fresh thyme stems (chopped)
Sprinkle with soy sauce or coconut aminos (to taste)
Olive oil

Coat a glass baking dish with olive oil. Place the salmon in the dish. Rub the olive oil on the top of the fish. After coating the top of the salmon with the olive oil, turn it over so the skin side is down. Chop up the fresh herbs and place in a bowl. Add the sliced black olives on top of the fish. Sprinkle the fresh cut herbs on top of the olives. Drizzle a little soy sauce or coconut aminos over the top. Bake the salmon in the oven for 20 minutes. Serve right out of the oven alone or with other side items.

Homemade Salsa

5-6 large ripe tomatoes
1 large red onion
2-3 cayenne peppers (chopped)
1-2 cloves fresh garlic
1/2 fresh lime (juiced)
cilantro
salt
pepper

Wash 5-6 large tomatoes. If you use smaller ones, you will need to use a few more. Using a large knife, chop the tomatoes into small chunks and place in a large bowl. Next you will need 1 large red onion or several smaller ones. Chop the onion into small, diced chunks and add on top of the tomatoes. If you like your salsa hot, you will need to add several cayenne peppers. Chop the cayenne peppers into small, diced pieces and add on top of the tomatoes and onion. Next you will want to add your fresh garlic to a garlic press and squeeze it into the bowl of prepared chopped vegetables. Chop some fresh cilantro (use about a handful from the bunch) and add it to the other vegetables. Next take your lime and cut it in half. Squeeze the juice from half of the lime on top of the vegetable mix. Add your salt and pepper and any other seasonings you may like on top and then stir the vegetables together. Season the mix to taste. Stir until vegetables are well mixed. Serve with chips, crackers, bread or an entrée.

Skinny Chicken and Broccoli Alfredo

3 boneless, skinless chicken breasts, cut into chunks (about 2 cups)
2 cups fresh broccoli florets
1-8 oz. package fresh mushrooms (sliced)
1 small onion (chopped)
8 oz. whole grain fettuccine or other favorite noodle
(you can find one made from chick peas if you can't eat gluten)
2 tbsp. extra virgin olive oil
2 tsp. minced garlic
2 tbsp. flour or cornstarch
1-1/2 to 2 cups chicken broth
1/2 cup plain Greek yogurt
1/2 cup skim milk, almond milk or cashew milk
Salt and pepper to taste (add in any other spices you like)
Crushed red pepper to taste
3/4 cup freshly grated Parmesan cheese

In a pot of boiling water, cook the pasta according to package directions. Drain and set aside.

In a medium frying pan, heat the olive oil over medium-low heat. Add the chicken and garlic and sauté until the chicken is browned, stirring frequently. Add the broccoli, onion and mushrooms and stir. Add the salt and pepper and crushed red pepper and any other spices that sound good to you. Next, gradually whisk in the chicken broth, Greek yogurt and milk. Whisk in the flour until smooth, about 2 minutes. Bring to a low boil, stirring constantly. Lower the heat and simmer for several minutes. Stir in the Parmesan cheese.

Serve over prepared noodles. Add butter or olive oil to the noodles to coat, before serving, if desired. Add additional Parmesan to the top, if desired. Serve with a healthy side salad if you like to add in some additional vegetables and nutrients to your meal.

Stuffed Peppers

4-6 large green peppers
12 oz. pork sausage (you can substitute hamburger or ground turkey)
2/3 cup chopped red onion
1/2 package (4 oz.) fresh sliced mushrooms
1/3 cup thinly sliced celery
1 cup diced fresh tomatoes (you can also substitute diced canned tomatoes or a good quality pasta sauce)
1 small can sliced olives
2 fresh cloves of garlic (crushed)
1 cup cooked rice (choose your favorite variety)
1 egg (beaten)
1/2 tsp. salt
1/4 tsp. pepper
Cajun seasoning to taste
1-8 oz. package grated cheddar cheese

Cut tops off peppers and scrape out seeds. Boil some water in a large pot (enough to cover peppers) and add the peppers, boiling for approximately 5 minutes to cook slightly. Remove from heat, rinse and drain to cool.

Cook the pork sausage in a large skillet over medium heat, stirring frequently to break up the meat. Add the onion, celery, olives, mushrooms, garlic, salt, pepper and Cajun seasoning, stirring occasionally until the sausage is cooked through and the vegetables are tender. Transfer the sausage mixture into a large mixing bowl and allow it to cool slightly. Add the diced tomatoes and egg. Add the rice to the cooled sausage mixture and scoop into the peppers. Sprinkle grated cheese over the top of the peppers. Bake until the peppers are tender and crisp in a 350 degree oven for approximately 30 minutes.

Best Black Bean Salsa

1 15 oz. can black beans (drained)
1 16 oz. can corn (drained)
1 red bell pepper (diced)
1 green bell pepper (diced)
1 yellow bell pepper (diced)
1/2 cup red onion (diced)
1 garlic clove (minced)
1 tsp. cilantro
1/4 cup olive oil
4 tbsp. red wine vinegar
1 tsp. lime juice
Freshly ground pepper
Salt
Tortilla chips

Seed and dice the bell peppers. In a salad bowl, combine bell peppers, onion, corn kernels, garlic and cilantro. Toss to mix. Add black beans, olive oil, vinegar and lime juice. Salt and pepper the mix to taste. Toss again. Serve with tortilla chips.

Note: If corn is in season, you can use fresh corn. Use 1 or 2 ears. You will need to cut it off the cob.

Easy Fruit and Cream Cheese Squares

Crust
2 cups crushed almonds
1/2 cup coconut oil (melted)

Filling
1 package cream cheese (8 oz.)
6 oz. high-quality chocolate chips (look for high cacao content)
1/4 cup raw honey

Topping
blueberries
cherries (remove pits)

Using a food processor, crush almonds and pour in a large bowl. Add the melted coconut oil and stir until it is thoroughly mixed with the crushed almonds. Press the almond mixture into a greased 8" x 8" or 9" x 9" pan. Bake for 10 minutes. Remove from oven to cool. Melt the chocolate chips. Spread them over the cooled crust. Let the chocolate mixture harden. (To speed up the process, put the pan in the refrigerator for an hour.) In the meantime, in a mixer, add the cream cheese and honey and mix well. Spread the mixture over the hardened chocolate crust. Top the mixture with blueberries and cherries and chill for a few hours.

Note: You can use any other fruit toppings you like.

Chocolate Cream Caramel Bars

Crust
2 cup walnuts
2 cup dates
Pinch of salt (optional)

Caramel
1 cup cashew butter or almond butter
1 cup coconut oil
2 cup dates

Chocolate Cream
2/3 cup coconut oil
5-6 tbsp. cacao powder
1/2 cup honey

To make the crust: process the nuts into a flour mix in your food processor, then add the dates and process until it all begins to stick together. Press into the bottom of a 9" x 9" glass baking dish.

To make both the caramel and mocha layers: blend the ingredients in each list until smooth. Spread the caramel onto your crust, followed by the chocolate cream. Refrigerate until completely set (this will take a couple hours). You can also place the pan in the freezer to speed up the process for each layer.

ABOUT THE AUTHOR

Barbara Rodgers is a certified health coach and former small business owner.

With her training at Institute of the Integrative Nutrition®, she understands how the mind, body and spirit are all interconnected and play an integral part in our overall health.

Barbara loves to cook and bake. Growing up, she enjoyed being in the kitchen and has vivid memories of helping prepare meals. This is where she developed an enthusiasm for cooking and baking for family and friends. While she always had an interest in nutrition and exercise, it wasn't until she developed an iron deficiency a few years ago that her interest in nutrition turned into a passion.

Barbara uses this passion to connect and help others going through changes and challenges—especially women at mid-life—feel balanced and alive again. She takes pleasure in spending time with her family and enjoys time at the lake. She likes to write, blog, read, walk, do yoga, play tennis, water ski, hula hoop and jump on the trampoline.

Connect With Barbara!

barbararodgersonline.com

brodgers483@gmail.com

Instagram: @barb.rodgers
Facebook: Barbara Rodgers Health Coach

RESOURCES

[1]"Carrie H., Age 56." Women to Women. N.p., 12 Nov. 2014. Web. 31 Jan. 2017.
https://www.womentowomen.com/menopause-perimenopause/perimenopause/

[2]"Wpadmin. "22 Shocking Iron Deficiency Anemia Statistics." HRFnd. N.p., 23 Dec. 2014. Web. 01 Feb. 2017.

[3]Mayo Clinic Staff Print. "Iron Deficiency Anemia." Overview - Iron Deficiency Anemia - Mayo Clinic. N.p., 11 Nov. 2016. Web. 13 Feb. 2017.

[4]Mayo Clinic Staff Print. "Ferritin Test." Results - Ferritin Test - Mayo Clinic. N.p., 29 Nov. 2016. Web. 14 Dec. 2016.
http://www.mayoclinic.org/tests-procedures/ferritin-test/details/results/rsc-20271960

[5]"Overweight and Obesity Statistics." National Institutes of Health. U.S. Department of Health and Human Services, n.d. Web. 16 Jan. 2017.

[6]Buettner, Dan. "Chapter 4." The Blue Zones Solution: Eating and Living like the World's Healthiest People. N.p.: n.p., n.d. N. pag. Print. (Loc. 807 on Kindle)

[7]Buettner, Dan. "Chapter 4." The Blue Zones Solution: Eating and Living like the World's Healthiest People. N.p.: n.p., n.d. N. pag. Print. (Loc. 64, 77, 183, 214, 225, 240 on Kindle)

[8]"Food Fortification." Wikipedia. Wikimedia Foundation, n.d. Web. 12 May 2016.

[9]"Food Fortification." Wikipedia. Wikimedia Foundation, n.d. Web. 12 May 2016.

[10]"Why Food Fortification. PHC Project Healthy Children." N.p., n.d. Web.

[11]"Food Fortification." Wikipedia. Wikimedia Foundation, n.d. Web. 12 May 2016.

[12] Wpadmin. "22 Shocking Iron Deficiency Anemia Statistics." HRFnd. N.p., 23 Dec. 2014. Web. 01 Feb. 2017.

[13]Rosenthal, Joshua. "Notes from IIN's Founder: Why It's OK to Quit Being Vegan or Macrobiotic." Institute For Integrative Nutrition. N.p., n.d. Web.

[14]Rosenthal, Joshua. "Post Modern Nutrition." Integrative Nutrition Feed Your Hunger For Health & Happiness. N.p.: Greenleaf Book LLC, 2014. 37-41. Print.

[15] "Iron We Consume." Idi. N.p., n.d. Web. 16 Dec. 2016. http://www.irondisorders.org/iron-we-consume/

[16]"Top Iron-Rich Foods List." WebMD. WebMD, n.d. Web. 13 Jan. 2017. http://www.webmd.com/diet/iron-rich-foods#1

[17]Permutter, David. Grain Brain: The Surprising Truth about Wheat, Carbs and Sugar--Your Brain's Silent Killers. N.p.: n.p., n.d. 62. Print.

[18]"Genetically Modified Food." Wikipedia. Wikimedia Foundation, n.d. Web. 27 Dec. 2016.

[19]"Healthy, Brightly Colored Vegetables." LIVESTRONG.COM. LIVESTRONG.COM, 16 Aug. 2013. Web. 15 Sept. 2016.

[20]"10 Antioxidant Super Foods." WebMD. WebMD, n.d. Web. 21 Sept. 2016.

[21]60 Minutes Documentary Titled, "Is Sugar Toxic," Dr. Robert Lustig,. N.p., n.d. Web.

[22]"Dr. Mark Hyman On Sugar & The Only Rules You Need To Eat Healthy."Mindbodygreen. N.p., 13 June 2014. Web. 03 June 2016. http://www.mindbodygreen.com/.

[23]"Processed Foods History: 1910s to 1950s." Modern Pioneer Mom. N.p., 05 July 2012. Web. 31 Jan. 2017.

[24]"How Many Teaspoons of Sugar Are There in a Can of Coke?" LIVESTRONG.COM. Leaf Group, 14 Apr. 2015. Web. 31 Jan. 2017.

[25]"Caramel Frappuccino® Blended Coffee." Starbucks Coffee Company. N.p., n.d. Web. 31 Jan. 2017.

[26]CNN. Cable News Network, n.d. Web. 31 Jan. 2017. http://www.cnn.com/2014/08/07/health/restaurant-fast-food-calories/

[27] Ewg. "EWG's 2017 Shopper's Guide to Pesticides in Produce." EWG. N.p., n.d. Web. 17 Mar. 2017. http://www.ewg.org/foodnews

[28]Ewg. "EWG's 2017 Shopper's Guide to Pesticides in Produce." EWG. N.p., n.d. Web. 17 Mar. 2017. http://www.ewg.org/foodnews

[29]"Community Supported Agriculture." Community Supported Agriculture - LocalHarvest. N.p., n.d. Web. 01 Feb. 2017.

[30]"Integrative Nutrition: Feed Your Hunger for Health & Happiness." Issuu. N.p., n.d. Web. 01 Feb. 2017.

[31]Mathew Kelly. Becoming the Best Version of Yourself. Beacon Publishing, 1999. CD.

[32]Brian Johnson's Philosophers Notes—Clean. http://www.entheos.com/philosophersnotes/notes/all/Clean, pg. 2

[33]"Hippocrates Quote." A-Z Quotes. N.p., n.d. Web. 20 Mar. 2017.

[34] "Auguste Comte Quote." A-Z Quotes. N.p., n.d. Web. 20 Mar. 2017.

[35]"Leigh Hunt Quote." A-Z Quotes. N.p., n.d. Web. 20 Mar. 2017.

[36]"Leonardo Da Vinci Quote." A-Z Quotes. N.p., n.d. Web. 20 Mar. 2017.

[37]"John Ruskin Quote." A-Z Quotes. N.p., n.d. Web. 20 Mar. 2017.

[38]"Pablo Picasso Quote." A-Z Quotes. N.p., n.d. Web. 20 Mar. 2017.

[39]"Voltaire Quote." A-Z Quotes. N.p., n.d. Web. 20 Mar. 2017.

[40]"Mahatma Gandhi Quote." A-Z Quotes. N.p., n.d. Web. 20 Mar. 2017.